Apple Cider Vinegar

Holistic Apple Cider Vinegar Recipes & Uses for Health, Beauty & Cooking

By Cassia Albinson

Copyright © Cassia Albinson 2016

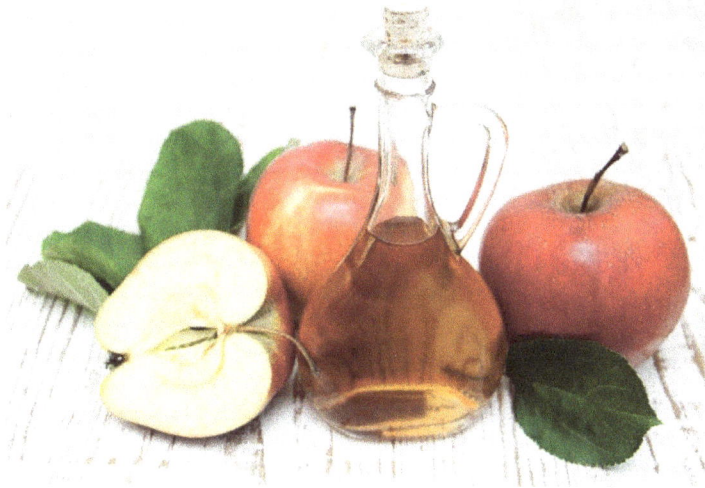

Contents

Introduction 8

Chapter 1 – History of Apple Cider Vinegar (ACV)........................10

ACV and Fermentation 10

Fermentation, Nutrition, and Digestion.................................. 11

History of Apple Cider Vinegar...12

Wines, Vinegars and ACV 13

Types of ACV 15

Kombucha v ACV 17

Chapter 2 ACV and Health 18

Digestion & Weight Loss...19

Diabetes...21

Bloating 22

Reflux/Heartburn 22

Waste Removal... 23

Heart Support 24

Nausea 25

Detoxing 26

Sinuses...27

Skin... 28

Itches, Scratches, Bites and Stings 28

Sunburn... 29

Wart Remover 29

Acne 30

Nail Fungus and Athletes Foot 30

Smelly Feet 31

Wound Cleaning... 32

Hives & Shingles 32

Hemorrhoids.. 33

Cold Sores + Vitamin C 33

Metabolism 33

Nervous System 34

Ears 35

Hiccups 35

Muscles 35

Dental/Oral.. 36

General Infections and Viruses 36

Sore Throats.. 37

Circulation 37

Cancer Caution 38

Chapter 3 ACV and Cooking................................... 40

Smoothies 40

Casseroles 41

Sauces 41

Soups.. 42

Salads 42

Chapter 4 – Apple Cider Vinegar and Beauty 43

Hair 43

Dandruff... 44

Removal of Nits/Lice... 44

Skin 44

To Ease Out Blackheads 45

Acne 46

Aftershave 47

Age spots 47

Warts 47

Sunburns 48

Fades Bruises 49

Chapter 5 - ACV in the Home 50

First Aid 51

Kitchen Cleaning 51

Drains 52

Washing Machine 52

Steam Iron 52

Appliances 53

Cutting Boards 53

Fridge/Freezer 53

Ice Trays 53

Kettles etc. 54

Bottles 54

Bathroom 54

Makeup Brushes 55

Toothbrush holder 55

Bathroom Ceramics 56

Shower Cubicle 56

Dining Room 56

Lounge 56

Wood Scratches 57

Office 57

Patio 58

Garden Furniture 58

Garden 58

Chapter 6 - Making your own ACV 60

Goodbye and Good Natural Health...............................63

Introduction

Welcome to the fascinating world of Apple Cider Vinegar (ACV).

You may have noticed over the last year or two in magazines, health blogs, and Facebook that Apple Cider Vinegar (ACV) has been getting a lot of good press. Many claims are being made for how effective it is and these range from a cure for cancer – all the way through to stopping smelly feet!

Quite rightly people get suspicious when so many claims are being made and wonder just what they can rely on – and what they need to ignore as 'the latest craze.' It always sounds exciting when you read that first article, but by the time you get to the third, fourth and fifth the excitement tends to give way to cynicism.

This book has been written to reassure you and warn you.

Yes, some of the claims that have been made are wild! They are not tested and verified.

Yes, some of the claims are correct and have stood the test of time.

This book will tell you what to trust, when to use common sense and when to steer clear.

That being said, ACV has many uses – and a long history - so it is definitely something to inform yourself about.

In this book, we will look first at the history of ACV and begin to understand how it came into being. However we will also look at the various vitamins, minerals, enzymes &microflora that are in ACV so that you will figure out why it does what it does, and when to be suspicious of some claims.

We will then look at the many ways it can be used to support your Health, and that of your family.

That will be followed by a chapter on using it for beauty purposes, where it can be very lovely to use for some tasks.

Next, up, we will look at how to use it in the home to keep that healthy and beautiful too!

Finally, there is a recipe for making your own ACV which is four times cheaper than buying the good stuff in the local health food store. You're going to enjoy that one.

You can use this book to get yourself up to date on all aspects of ACV, or you can just concentrate on the section that you are most interested in. Of course, the best way to learn about anything is by trying it out yourself and if that is the way you like to learn then I advise you to go and buy a couple of bottles of raw, unpasteurized ACV from your local store. Put one in the bathroom and one in the kitchen and then skim through the health, beauty and home chapters for a few ideas. Then just try it! You'll soon find out if it works for you. And you will have some fun!

Enjoy this journey into the fresh, zingy world of Apple Cider Vinegar...

Chapter 1 – History of Apple Cider Vinegar (ACV)

Amazingly ACV has been around for thousands of years! The reason for this is because it is the product of a process called fermentation.

ACV and Fermentation

Fermentation is a process which transforms one type of matter into another. You might recognise it as the process that changes a lovely fresh apple (or any kind of food, or wood or living matter) from a state of freshness all the way through to a decayed piece of 'something' a month later.

The agents of fermentation are microscopic bacteria, fungi, yeasts and molds which are floating in the air we breathe, the surfaces we touch and the food we eat. These microflora, as all the components are called, land on the fresh matter and begin to digest and change it from one form to another. For example, from juice to alcohol – to vinegar.   More on this in a minute as I tell you about the coming of apple cider vinegar itself!

Fermentation, Nutrition, and Digestion

These microflorae are an essential part of our health and our lives as they work with our guts to process food and drink in ways that make them more nutritious for us. You have probably been eating many fermented products all of your life. Think – cheese, bread, chocolate, coffee, wine, beer and vinegar! All of these fermentation products have distinctive tastes and flavors which give us so many delicacies in every culture of the world.

Fermentation makes our food more digestible, tastier and more nutritious. This is because the minerals and vitamins, trace elements and proteins in the food can be more readily absorbed once they have been 'worked on' by the microflora that makes fermentation happen.

In our culture, we wage a war against bacteria, fungi, and microbes, swiping and swabbing them away with antibacterial and antiseptic wipes. But in fact, we would be healthier if we exposed ourselves a little more to the raw, live and unpasteurized foods and drinks created by fermentation. We would be working in harmony with a natural process then. In fact, we are already in a symbiotic relationship with these microorganisms in our guts, on our skin and in the air around us.

Astonishingly we are actually their descendants. Every form of life on earth comes from micro bacteria when we look at fossil records. That is quite a thought!

History of Apple Cider Vinegar

Way back in Egyptian times vinegars were used for preserving, pickling, dissolving and flavoring. Ancient ceramics show traces of vinegars in the remains. Later the Samurai in Japan regularly took Egg Vinegar to give them strength. They made this by steeping a raw egg (with the shell on) in vinegar for a week. During this time the shell is dissolved and the remaining yolk, membrane and albumen are then stirred into the calcium rich vinegar and taken in doses of 5-10mls/day. That's about 1- 2 teaspoons. The Samurai lifestyle was demanding, and they certainly had to have stamina and power to survive it so perhaps it was that Egg Nog that did the trick.

Moving forward in time to the ancient Greeks and the father of medicine himself, Hippocrates, around 300BC. We find him prescribing vinegars for many ills including headaches, tummy aches and putting it on wounds.

The Ancient Persians caught onto the use of vinegar and a weight control support and drank it regularly to manage their body fat.

The Romans, such as Hannibal in his famous march across the Alps, used hot vinegar like dynamite to dissolve and splinter the rocks. This cleared the way for his troops and elephants to move through the mountains.

Later still it was used in many wars, right through to World War I – from cleaning chain mail with a scoop of sand made into a paste with vinegar in medieval times to being the disinfectant used on the battlefields of France.

Wines, Vinegars and ACV

So vinegars, in general, have a long and venerable history mainly because vinegars (from whatever vegetable or fruit it is made) have many properties. They dissolve, flavor, energise, disinfect, preserve, control sugar intake, supply enzymes, and trace elements to give just a few examples.

But what about ACV itself? Vinegars began as the last part of a fermentation process which started with a fruit or a grain. So we made wine from grapes, beer from grain and even a sour apple wine from the Phoenicians which was the forerunner of our cider from apples. All ancient apples were very sour, like our crab apples, and only as the farming community began to experiment with size and flavour of apples did the large sweet apples appear or the sharper varieties emerge. Wine turns into vinegar if left exposed to air – and so vinegar was born.

So from the early 17th Century when apples were harvested in the early autumn, and crisp apple juice was pressed from the fibrous fruit the making of cider became a commercial process. In fact, if you leave any fruit juice in a wide mouthed container, covered with a piece of cheesecloth you will find it turns into alcohol. It does this is as short a time as a week. With apples, this is hard cider, which doesn't have much fizz. Leaving it a bit longer as the microflora in the air start to have a yeast action on the liquid and carbon is released and the fizzy varieties emerge. Leave it longer still – another 4 weeks – and the alcohol will have turned to vinegar (acetic acid). That is the final product of the fermentation process and bringing that apple cider vinegar into the kitchen means you can cook with it by using it as a condiment and as a preservative as you pickle fresh fruit and vegetables to store them for winter.

Or you can use it as a medicine by drinking it regularly (more on that later as it is important to take the right amount and have the level of dilution correct.) You can also use it in combination with other healthy herbs, spices, and oils to create home remedies to support everyday ailments.

Alternatively take it into the bathroom or pop it into the cupboard under the sink and you can use it in a variety of ways as a household cleanser and beauty aid. Much more on these three ways to use ACV later in the following chapters.

Types of ACV

There various types of apple cider vinegar you can get when you go to the shops:

Pasteurized or unpasteurized. Pasteurizing heats up the ACV and renders it inert so that it is fine for flavoring or cleaning, but not for using as a health boost. For the health boost, you need raw, unpasteurized ACV where the good micro bacteria, enzymes, and trace elements remain and these will work in conjunction with your own body systems to help support and heal.

Raw ACV also means it is unpasteurized and that it contains the 'mother' which is like a floating raft of beneficial microflora eating up the sugar and alcohol in the cider and turning it into acetic acid. The 'mothers,' or SCOBY's (Symbiotic Culture of Bacteria and Yeast) look rather alarming – a thin, almost transparent disc of gelatinous mass – like a jellyfish!   But in fact, this is a marvelous miracle of Nature and is extremely good for us. It will make the ACV in your bottle look a bit cloudy, and you will see small trails of matter drifting through the liquid. This is a good sign that the fermentation process has worked, and the liquid that is left is no longer alcoholic.

Filtered or Unfiltered – this means that the bits and pieces of apple matter and the 'mother' have been filtered out – or not. Again, the unfiltered variety is far better for health purposes. The filtered variety is fine for flavoring.

Organic – this means that the original apples in the juice and cider stages were farmed organically without chemical insecticides or biochemical fertilizers. For health reasons organic is definitely superior.

ACV contains vitamins, minerals such as boron, iron, potassium and magnesium and other micronutrients all of which have a part to play in supporting a healthy body.

The last part of the story of ACV

Did you know about Switchels?

Let's finish off this journey through history and the uses of fermentation, vinegars and particularly ACV, with some last little 'take-aways.'

Mainly ACV is used for flavoring purposes and as a health aid. However, it is also lovely as an ingredient in a different drink. This drink is called a Switchel and is a combination of ACV and something rich, dark, sweet and flavorsome like molasses and something spicy and hot like ginger root. This can be used as a restorative tonic and is mighty nice! Switchels can be made with a variety of other ingredients along with ACV. You are only limited by your imagination.

Kombucha v ACV

For those of you who know about Kombucha, there are many similarities between the two regarding their properties, but there are also differences in the microflora that act as the fermenting agents. Kombucha can still have alcohol in the final liquid (very, very little), whereas ACV does not have any. Kombucha is made with the herb, tea, rather than a fruit like apples. The taste varies between the two with ACV being quite sharp and Kombucha being more mellow – but much depends on how long they have been left to ferment to the final stage. Old ACV and old Kombucha are both STRONG tasting.   There are more beneficial enzymes and biochemicals in Kombucha than ACV. ACV is acetic acid in the end, and Kombucha has a variety of organic acids. Kombucha can also be added to fruit, molasses, honey, ginger, etc. to make it more palatable.

Chapter 2 ACV and Health

So let's look now at the health benefits of ACV. There are so many it is very exciting to see. One glimpse in Google and you will reel with the lists you will find. However, this is where there have been some big claims made and where it is most sensible to read up carefully and make your own judgements.

As you can tell from the description of ACV in the last chapter the properties of this liquid mean, it can be a useful friend in many circumstances. In particular, it's antiseptic, antibiotic, anti-inflammatory, antioxidant, anti-fungal and alkalizing properties help in many aspects of health.

- ✓ Antiseptic - prevents the growth of disease-causing micro-organisms, gives a deep clean and sterilizes
- ✓ Antibiotic – inhibits growth and spread of specific microorganisms
- ✓ Anti-inflammatory - acts to reduce swelling, tenderness, fever, redness
- ✓ Anti-oxidant - prevents the start of a chain reaction of biochemical events as oxygen combines with elements which can disrupt the integrity of cells
- ✓ Anti-fungal - prevents the spread of mold spores and fungi

✓ Alkalinizing - changes the pH of the system. e.g., acidosis caused by kidney problems or diet.

This section is split into the different systems and functions of the body and shows you how to use ACV in each to help you to better health.

Digestion & Weight Loss

Here ACV is a hero in many ways.

Speeds up your digestion.

Firstly it helps by encouraging the breakdown of food particles as the food reaches the stomach. To do this, you need to have one of your daily doses of ACV before you eat.

Dosage:

Take this as a daily drink starting with no more than 1 teaspoonful/glass of water twice a day. Take this before you eat. Use a highball sized glass so the ACV is well diluted.

 Gradually increase this to 3 times/day. Give yourself at least a week to get used to the dosage. If your body feels happy....go on to the next increase.

After another week or two, and only if your body is responding well, increase this to 1 dessertspoon/glass 3 times/day.

After another week or two and depending how your body is responding increase this to 1 tablespoon in a glass of water 3x/day.

Make sure the ACV contains the 'mother' or SCOBY that we discussed in the previous chapter. You can do this by shaking the bottle before you pour. All you need is a smidgeon of the cloudiness the live enzymes and yeasts cause, and it gives a wonderful boost to your system.

ACV helps in weight control.

It does this by making you have the sensation of being full so that your brain sends signals of 'satisfaction' and tells your body to stop eating. Partly this is achieved through having the dose before you eat so that the liquid contributes to the sensation of fullness, but the ACV itself also helps by curbing sugar conversion of the starches in the carbohydrates you have eaten.

Pasta lovers – pay attention! If you are having a high carbohydrate meal, it helps to have your pre-meal glass of ACV and water. It can mean that you eat around 250 calories less than you otherwise would have.

Remember to keep checking your body for the message that you are full. Often we miss that message and continue to eat out of habit. However, we are eating when we are not actually hungry. A study showed that a weight management plan which included the diluted dosage of 2x 1 tablespoon of ACV daily led to 2 kilos of weight loss. This took place over 12 weeks so it looks like ACV is a good friend alongside sensible lifestyle/diet choices.

Diabetes

This takes us to Diabetic support as ACV helps people who have diabetes by lowering LDL and A1C levels after meals. However, there has not been a great deal of research on this. If you are taking your daily dose of ACV and you find that your blood sugar levels are steadier this is a bonus. However, never increase the dosage to more than 3 tablespoons per day, well diluted with water.

If you have a history of kidney stones or stomach ulcers, you would be better to steer clear completely or to limit your daily dosage to just 1 teaspoon twice/day in order to enjoy the other benefits of ACV.

Please do not increase it and do not replace any medication you may have been given by the doctor. As always your body will be your guide and if you feel well and balanced on your ACV dosage stay with it. If you do not, or your reaction changes, stop immediately and do not continue with until you have seen your doctor and your body has settled down.

Bloating

This is when you feel uncomfortable; puffed up and a bit swollen around the tummy and midriff. It is often to do with a change in eating habits, such as having too much lactose, yeast or gluten when these are things you are a little sensitive to. There can be quite a lot of gas trapped in the digestive tract, and this needs to be reduced by releasing it by burping or passing wind.

ACV comes to the rescue again by changing the pH levels in the digestive tract and making it easier to break down the food particles you are sensitive to. As they dissolve and disperse into the system more quickly, there is less time for the body to react to their presence and build up gas.

By the way, if you hate, hate, hate the taste of ACV in your glass of water try using warm water and drizzling in a teaspoon of honey to change the taste. Use local honey so you also get a chance to change your sensitivity to the pollens that might be around.

Reflux/Heartburn

Indigestion has several causes, and it is always best to have this checked out if it is something you suffer from regularly. However, ACV is very useful for heartburn when it is caused by an under acidic condition in the stomach. A tablespoon of ACV in a large glass of water can speedily help the tummy regulate again and settle down. However, if you suffer from indigestion regularly, please do get it checked out.

Waste Removal

ACV's capacity to change and balance the pH of the system is a great benefit in many ways.

A body which is too acidic generally starts to struggle to process and absorb all the nutrients it needs from the food it is being given. Diets rich in red meats and too few green vegetables are very prone to being over-acidic. This can begin to affect the flushing function of the kidneys.

ACV can also help to get rid of any infection in the urinary tract through its antibiotic function. Just one glass of diluted ACV/day helps with both of these complaints.

However, I'm also going to pop in a gentle plea to consider adding more green vegetables to your diet! These help in many ways but mainly through providing a power pack of micronutrients in the form of trace elements and a boost of fiber to enable your bowel movements to be regular and the whole digestive tract cleansed. Truly, Mom was right. Eat your greens!

Heart Support

Since heart disease is one of the biggest causes of death, it is important to maintain a healthy heart. If you have already got the symptoms of heart disease such as high or fluctuating, Blood Pressure there are several studies pointing to a daily dose of ACV being beneficial in reducing some of the symptoms.

Lowers cholesterol

First of all, it can lower cholesterol levels. High cholesterol levels are thought to increase the risk of heart disease so a daily routine that keeps the levels under control, along with a sensible diet can be a great way to look after your heart.

Lowers Triglycerideide levels

Second, ACV lowers triglyceride levels which help to stop fat accumulating and blood pressure rising. Studies are pointing to triglycerides causing thickening of the artery walls, and this not only increases blood pressure but also increases the risk of having a stroke or a heart attack. Well worth keeping your triglycerides low - and these can be determined by a blood test if you are not sure what is happening in your body. Just ask your doctor.

Anti-oxidant

Third, the anti-oxidant properties of ACV help to protect LDL cholesterol from oxidizing. By doing this, the chain reaction of changes in the cells of the particles is halted, and the cholesterol levels stay safe with none of the dangers of inflammation happening.

Try this to lower your Cholesterol level.

Make one of your daily doses of ACV into a delicious drink.

Take an apple, some grapes and 1 tablespoon of ACV in a tall glass of water. Blend them all in the blender to make a smoothie and enjoy.

Nausea

This can happen if you have had food that doesn't agree with you and which contains some very unfriendly bacteria! It's the body's way of protecting us by getting rid of what is unsafe for the whole system.

One of the great qualities of the skin is that much that is beneficial can be absorbed through it so for nausea and vomiting making a warm compress out of a towel or a washcloth and soaking it in ACV is very soothing and healing.

Dosage: Use 1 liter of warm water and 300 ml of ACV. Soak the washcloth in it and gently squeeze out the excess liquid so that it doesn't run down your body and pool underneath you. Lie down and just rest as the body soaks up the goodness. You can replace the warm washcloth three times over a 20 minute period, and you should fell much better after that.

ACV is a very effective detoxing agent. It can be used to do this in several ways. First, it depends whether the detox you want is for an overall 'flush out' of the remains in the body at the end of a season and in getting ready for the next one. Or, is it for something specific like breaking up mucus and easing sinus congestion because of infection following a cold.

Detoxing

If it is the first, the way to get going is by reviewing your current 'not so helpful habits.' This is a polite way of saying are you eating too many carbs, sugars, and fats? Have you let your exercise regime slip a bit because of busyness - or habit? Think of the diet that suits your metabolism best from past experience and also consider what light exercise do you enjoy most. Make the decision that you will commit to this detox and START! Your ACV will support the other aspects and make them far more effective.

Dosage: Take 12 ounces of warm filtered water add 4 tablespoons each of ACV with the mother, pure lemon juice, and local raw honey. Add a sprinkle of cinnamon and a dash of cayenne pepper to you taste. You can also pop in a slice of apple to give you some fiber. Drink slowly before a light meal and enjoy. Do this for 5 days and feel pepped up and ready for the next season.

If it is the second way just keep up with your daily routine of a glass of ACV mixture before each meal and use ACV compresses on your chest, nose and cheeks to break up the mucus and allow it to disperse and drain.

Sinuses

Your sinuses can become infected and blocked due to having had a cold or flu which has dragged on. This is exactly when you need to go back to the ancient, yogic technique of 'neti.'

Dosage: This involves sniffing a cup of warmed water mixed with a half teaspoon of ACV. Just tilt the cup, or pour a bit of diluted ACV into your hand and snort it up into one nostril while you hold the other one closed with a finger. Sounds complicated but it's not when you do it! Hold your head back, then to one side, then the other. Unplug your closed nostril and let the liquid just run out of both. Then do the same on the other side.

You may find your nose drips for a while after - so have your tissues handy – as it is very prone to just suddenly start dripping when you are not expecting it!

The antibacterial effect of ACV will work on the accumulated mucus and break it up.

Skin

This is our next big area for some ACV help. The skin forms a wonderful protective covering over your body. Not only is it waterproof, but it is also porous. This means that it can be used as a medium to help us take in treatments of all kinds. The beneficial agents in the treatments - typically essential oils through massage, minerals, and vitamins through warm compresses or moisture through lotions and creams - all soak into the blood stream through the skin and are carried to the areas requiring them.

ACV can also be used as a specific remedy for areas of the skin which have been affected, infected or inflamed. As always you will use it in diluted form as the acetic acid it contains can be strong if it is applied in its pure form.

So, let us look at ways we can use those properties of ACV on various ailments afflicting the skin.

Itches, Scratches, Bites and Stings

This is a category of help where you need to carry around a small bottle of pre-diluted ACV in your bag and have it handy to apply when you are out and about in nature. Lovely as Nature is she can deliver some nasty bites and stings!

Even take ACV to the beach in case you or one of the family get stung by jellyfish. Those drifty tentacles they have can deliver a hefty wallop if they catch you as they float past. Water helps to sluice off the toxins, but the diluted ACV also helps to take down any inflammation.

Dosage: Just dampen a tissue or handkerchief with the ACV mixture and dab it on frequently until the irritation dies down. Dabbing on every 5/10 minutes works well depending on the intensity of the itch or sting.

Sunburn

While you are out in nature, you are also more likely to get sunburn unless you are very careful with your suncream application. There can easily just be one little spot you miss!

Your ACV mix as above will help to take the inflammation down once the worst happens! Just dab on regularly while the 'burn' dies down in the same way you did with the stings.

Wart Remover

Some people report having good results with using dilute ACV to remove warts and reduce or remove sunspots. The way it works is the acetic acid in the mixture removes cells and the wart or raised red cells from sun spots are gradually lessened.

Dosage: This needs daily application morning and night at a dilution of 2 parts water to 1 part ACV. As with the other applications just dab it on and let it dry naturally. This takes a few weeks to work - so it is worth persevering.

Acne

We have seen ACV's antiseptic and antibiotic effects already, and they can be used for outbreaks of acne too.

Dosage: It is extremely important that the ACV is diluted at the ratio of 3 parts water to 1 part ACV as you do not want to aggravate the skin tissue by using the harsh ACV on its own.

Just make up your solution and apply it morning and night. Watch for the infection in the pores to gradually reduce as the skin is kept clean and the deep cleanse works its way through the pores.

Nail Fungus and Athletes Foot

These are annoying, itchy conditions that definitely need the ACV touch.

Dosage: The easiest way to treat this is by making up a foot, or hand bath filled with warm dilute ACV (2 parts water to 1 part ACV) and soak twice/day.

If the nails have become particularly yellowed through the fungus, it is possible to use half a cup each of ACV and warm water (1:1) and soak in that mixture for 20 minutes before rinsing well.

Then rub in some olive oil to the nail bed. Do this twice/day until the yellowing fades and the nails are healthy.

Smelly Feet

While we are on the subject of feet, it is a good time to mention that ACV works well for reducing the smelly feet situation! Helpfully the ACV smell vanishes after a few minutes, but the effects of it continue!

Dosage: To reduce the condition if you or someone in the family suffer from this just soak as was recommended above in the 2 parts water to 1 part ACV dilution once/day.

It can also be extremely helpful for cases of fungus, athletes foot and smelly feet to wash the socks in a dilute mixture of ACV too. Soak them in the solution for half an hour before putting them through the normal wash cycle. That helps to stop any recurring infection take place.

Wound Cleaning

Talking of infections brings me to one of the best-known uses of ACV - in fact, it can be any kind of raw vinegar such as wine vinegar, rice vinegar or apple vinegar - when it is used as a swab for wounds. Its antiseptic properties go to work immediately protecting the open site from any infections entering the body. It has a long and venerable history on the battlefields to attest to its effectiveness as a cleanser and disinfectant.

Dosage: Use your 1 part ACV to 3 parts water for this.

Hives & Shingles

These are very irritating and painful conditions that can erupt on the skin. There are various causes, but the long and short of it is that they are extremely uncomfortable.

Dosage: Both respond well to an ACV bath where a warmish bath is run one-third full, and 500mls of ACV added. Soak in this for 20 minutes and repeat as often as you feel the need. 4 times/day is not unusual.

By the way, Psoriasis and eczema can be treated like this too.

Hemorrhoids

These are another painful and uncomfortable condition which make life unpleasant and diluted ACV can come to the rescue again.

Dosage: Just moisten a swab or piece of toilet paper with 3:1 water to ACV dilution and use that to dab onto the affected area. DO NOT USE ACV NEAT! You can imagine the stinging if you did.

Cold Sores + Vitamin C

Cold sores can be distressing to develop but if you increase your daily dose of Vitamin C (through eating more citrus fruit or taking the effervescent tablets from the chemist) and use dilute 1:3 ACV on the sore it will help it to dry up and heal more quickly.

Metabolism

Your metabolism is the process in you that dictates how quickly and effectively you absorb and use your food. This can vary according to all kinds of circumstances in your life. Diet, the level of exercise, age, and stress can all influence it. Fluctuations in your metabolism can make you feel very tired and fatigued. ACV helps to revive you by giving you an energy boost because it has potassium in it. It kicks up your low energy and helps to balance your metabolism if taken regularly.

Dosage: Just 1 teaspoon in a highball sized glass of water can help.

Taken nightly it will also help with insomnia.

However, if you take it as recommended earlier three times/day with food, you will find that it helps to lift your tiredness and even helps depression as well as supporting your metabolism generally.

Nervous System

Some people swear by ACV in dilution of 2 parts water to 1 part ACV for a headache cure. This can be administered as a vapor inhalation in just the same way as you might do with a Friar's Balsam or eucalyptus vapor bath for sinuses and cold relief.

Dosage: Half a teaspoon of ACV to a liter of hot water will give you some relief.

Ears

ACV can help the ears in two ways. First it is great for clearing ear infections, and second, it is good for clearing a blocked ear after swimming.

Dosage: Take your 3:1 dilution and using a dropper just drip 3 drops into the affected ear. Lie quietly for 5 minutes while it begins its work and repeat three times/day. If it persists for longer than 2 days, please go and see your doctor.

Hiccups

Hiccups can be relieved by taking a glass of dilute ACV and sipping gently to interrupt the spasms. It works even better if you try to drink from the opposite side of the glass! That takes your full attention and changes your breathing which then stops the hiccups!

Muscles

Nighttime leg cramps are usually to do with an imbalance of magnesium and/or potassium in the body.

Dosage: Taking a glass of 3:1 ACV before bed can relieve this annoying condition.

Dental/Oral

There is a lot of debate about using ACV to whiten your teeth. The acetic acid component means that it may well erode the tooth enamel if used frequently. To avoid this, it is recommended that you only use it as a whitener once/week and at a dilution of 3:1. Salt is an old remedy for this too and works well, but this also erodes enamel over time so using these with caution makes sense.

If you use the ACV dilution once/week, it will also help dispel bad breath and the vinegar smell will disappear very quickly.

General Infections and Viruses

Moving back to ACV as a friend for coughs and colds which involve viruses, bacteria and excess mucus you now know enough to think that there must be a way to use ACV for these conditions too. And there is. Take a washcloth, and as we did for the vomiting remedy, just soak it in warm, diluted ACV (3:1) and place it on your chest for 10 mins.

Dosage: Repeat this three or four times a day and take care to rest and drink plenty of water. That will keep the mucus more liquid and help you fight infection more quickly.

Sore Throats

For sore throats, you can use it more topically by gargling with your 3:1 dilution and let the solution absorb through your mouth tissue. Don't hold it in your mouth. Just gargling is enough.

Dosage: Do this for a couple of minutes twice/day. Morning and night.

Circulation

Poor circulation can also be part of a heart condition but if you find your legs aching for any reason making a warm compress to place over painful veins and just gently massaging the warmth and solution in while having your feet elevated can ease that heavy, uncomfortable achiness easily.

Dosage: Give yourself at least 20 minutes like this.

The other way to help yourself with this condition is to partly fill a bath with cold water, toss in 500mls ACV. Make sure the water covers your ankles and 'wade' up and down in the cool bath 10/12 times letting the water soothe your aches. Then go and lie down with your feet elevated and a soft towel around your feet and calves while the water dries off. Bliss.

Remember the daily remedy which will gently support your overall health:

1 teaspoon in large glass

Increase to 3 times/day

Increase to dessertspoon in large glass 3 x/day

Increase to one tablespoon in a large glass of water 3 x/day

Cancer Caution

A word of caution here because there is a buzz on the internet about using ACV as a cancer cure. However, the research has been done on rats or in test tubes and is not tested on humans at all. ACV seems to have some anti-cancerous properties such as shrinking tumors and killing cells and while it would be wonderful to think that this was a cure so readily available to all that is not a realistic claim at this time.

The other thing to bear in mind is that for truly lasting beneficial effects ACV needs to be part of a healthy lifestyle. This would include diet, exercise, mindfulness practices, etc. It is the holistic approach that works best to keep you in good shape or to support you through a time of ill health. One thing cannot have the same impact and ACV, or any one addition to your health care routine, is not a replacement for truly caring for yourself daily.

Chapter 3 ACV and Cooking

You can benefit very easily and quickly from all the health benefits in the last chapter by having your 1 - 3 daily doses of diluted ACV. However, a very pleasant way to get your daily dose is to make it a habit to add ACV to your cooking as well. This can be a great way to encourage the family to benefit too. Not many children like the tartness of a glass of diluted ACV so we turn to stealth and guile to work around this!

Here are some suggestions to start you off:

Smoothies

Smoothies are a great way to start of the day, or to have a healthy lunch on the move. They can be made with fruits or vegetables, or both. They can be 'beefed up' by adding milk to give them more protein, like a milkshake - or 'slimmed down' by adding filtered water/tomato juice or grapefruit juice and ACV. Remember that ACV helps you feel fuller!

Good mixtures to add to 2 tablespoons of ACV and 2 cups of water or juice are:

2 tablespoons of Cranberries

or

1 tablespoon of molasses

or

lemon and local honey

or

juiced carrot and celery

Pop the mixtures in a blender and whizz up to a good consistency. Add ice if you like it that way – and Enjoy.

Casseroles

Making a slow cook meal in the Crockpot? Add in that tablespoon of ACV to help balance any heaviness in the meat sauce.

Sauces

When you are reducing the juices in the pan to make your gravy or a sauce go with your roast, try popping in a tablespoon of ACV to balance out any over-saltiness.

If you are a fan - as I am - or delicious macaroni and cheese just try splashing in a tablespoon of ACV to the cheese sauce as you stir it when it is thickening. It gives it such a piquant lift.

Soups

Whether you are making a hearty winter soup with vegetables and beans or a light summery soup from stock and fresh vegetables a tablespoon of ACV will enhance the flavors and bring the digestive benefits of ACV straight to the table.

Salads

Salads are always improved by a dressing. Use Extra Virgin Olive oil or a creamy, lemony tasting avocado oil as the base ingredient and add ACV to make it pop. Even better add both a splash of ACV and a splash of fresh lemon juice to double the taste and benefits.

Chapter 4 – Apple Cider Vinegar and Beauty

Like many of the natural health supports such as Epsom Salt, honey and lemon juice ACV has uses as a beauty aid too. If you think of its properties - antiviral, antibiotic, antiseptic, antifungal, pH balancing, anti-inflammatory.. - you can quickly see ways it can be used in the bathroom as well as the kitchen.

It can be used internally and externally. Externally you can use it on wipes, or compresses as we did in the health chapter.
Internally it can be taken in a diluted form daily to support general health and bring a glow to your presence.

In the beauty world, it has two main uses. Hair and Skin. So let's take a look at how to use it for the best results.

Hair

Our crowning glory comes to life with an ACV rinse for the final sluice you give your hair after shampooing. This brightens the hair and makes it very shiny.

Amount: Take one-third of a cup ACV to 2 cups water.

Dandruff

This amount also helps control dandruff if you use it as your first rinse and massage in. Then rinse as normal.

Removal of Nits/Lice

For those awkward times when the children come home with some unwelcome visitors!

Shampoo and then apply the diluted ACV. Allow to remain on the hair for 10 mins then comb out with the special fine-toothed comb. It also seems to help if you add a drop of peppermint oil to the ACV mixture.

Amount: 1 cup ACV to 2 cups of water.

Skin

Kin is that wonderful organ of ours that is our first line of defense and protection. Our general health reflects through our skin, and we want it to be fresh, clean and glowing. This is where ACV come into its own.

First of all, it cleanses the skin.

You get a deep clean when used as part of your normal makeup removal and cleanse routine. Take a washcloth which has been soaked in a diluted mixture of ACV and water after you have used your regular products. Gently squeeze out the excess moisture and place the cloth over the face and allow it to moisten the skin and soak in. After the initial warmth of the cloth dies down make small, gentle circular movements with the cloth, thoroughly cleaning the whole of your face. This is also a good time to ease out any blackheads as the pores will be open, and the cleansing action of the ACV will be working.

Amount: 1 teaspoon ACV to 2 tablespoons of warm water.

To Ease Out Blackheads

The gentle circular movement you make with the washcloth will help to do this with blackheads that are near the surface of the skin.

Amount: For deeper blackheads try mixing 1 teaspoon Baking soda, 1 teaspoon ACV and 1 tablespoon water into a paste. Gently apply this paste to the affected area and leave until it dries. This acts as a facial mask. Clean it away with warm water and more gentle circles with a moist washcloth. This will help to break up and draw out the blackhead.

Acne

The same application works to help clear acne which needs a deep cleanse to help it heal. However, bear in mind that it is particularly important to have a high green vegetable and fiber diet while treating your acne as a great deal of help comes from 'internal' digestive support. Scrupulously clean skin and a healthy diet are the keys to acne removal.

Second, it balances the pH of the skin

Clean your skin as described above and while you do this, the ACV is working on balancing the acid and alkali levels in your skin. Our skin is at its best with a neutral level between the two.

Third, it tightens the skin.

After cleansing and balancing your skin, still using your washcloth, dip it again in a slightly weaker dilution of ACV and water. You can achieve this by adding another tablespoon of cold water to the liquid you had left after first soaking your washcloth. Soak your cloth again and wring out. Then wipe over your face. Doing this will tighten and tone your skin nicely.

You can also add a drop of your favorite essential oil to scent the ACV mixture. Do not use more than one drop in the dilution as pure essential oil is strong and could slightly burn your skin.

Aftershave

It is not only the ladies who can benefit from the ACV beauty bonuses. Men can use the 1:3 dilution as an aftershave astringent when it will tone and tighten the skin after shaving. It will close the pores and calm the skin.

Age spots

Remove age spots by applying a dab of diluted ACV daily. Just allow the dab to dry on the skin and the age spots will fade gradually. Don't expect a result overnight but keep it up and you will see a difference.

Amount: 1 part ACV: 2 parts water twice daily on the corner of a washcloth dabbed onto the skin.

Warts

Like age spots, warts can be eroded away through the cellular 'shrinking' and 'killing' properties of ACV. This also needs regular applications twice/day over some time. This time varies depending on how quickly the wart tissue takes to respond to the ACV.

Amount: Use as above for age spots.

Sunburns

Some sources claim that ACV calms down sunburn. This is one to try out for yourself as there seem to be two schools of thought. One that it works, and one that it doesn't! As long as you use a dilution of 1:3 (one ACV to three of water), you will be safe. What seems to vary is how effective it is.

There are different ways to apply it. You can fill a spray bottle and spray it on the affected areas, leaving it to dry naturally. Or you can put 2 cups of the diluted mixture in a cool bath and soak for ten minutes.

Either way, it is a good idea to apply some Aloe Vera cream as a moisturizer afterwards and let that re-hydrate the skin.

Fades Bruises

Bruises can be a bit unsightly if they are in an obvious place but ACV can come to the rescue again by helping them fade faster. A warm compress of 1:2 ACV and water, followed by a cold compress twice/day will bring the bruise to the surface and help it disperse into the network of capillaries more quickly. Use a washcloth or similar and leave the warm cloth on the skin until it cools. Then soak and wring out another cloth in cool ACV dilution and leave that on for 5 minutes.

Chapter 5 - ACV in the Home

It's ACV to the rescue again in the home. Instead of that 'chock-full of chemicals' bottle of bleach, you can make up a strong dilution of ACV and use that instead! In fact, it is a good idea once you are used to using ACV to make up 3 bottles of different dilutions and have them labelled and ready for use depending what you want to do. Make up one bottle with 1 part ACV to one part water. This is the strongest and only for use in cleaning the house. One part ACV to 2 parts water is more dilute and can be used in the home and for health and beauty support. One part ACV to 3 parts water is the most dilute and is used for health and beauty purposes.

If at any time, you feel the solution is too strong for your skin you can always dilute it even more by adding another 1 or 2 parts of water.

You are now ready to use it in the house. Remember how good it is as a cleaner, an odor neutralizer, disinfectant, and fungicide and you can start to imagine how many applications it has in the home!

First Aid

Along with the usual sticking plasters, bandages, scissors, and swabs keep a small spray bottle of diluted ACV (1:3) to spray on wounds, burns, bites or stings. It keeps for ages in a glass bottle so it is safe to leave it there. Do a refresh any time you use it or when you do your half yearly check on the kit. Don't use plastic spray bottles as the vinegar and the plastic will interact over time.

Now to ACV's huge range of cleaning applications. Sit back and be amazed there are MANY:

Kitchen Cleaning

Cleans fruit and vegetables when you drop in 3 tablespoons of ACV to your sink of warm water as you wash any fruit or vegetables you are about to use.

Cleans sticky scissors after snipping up all kinds of things which leave a sticky residue on the blades.

Drains

The drains outside the kitchen can become a bit smelly if food collects on the grid or grease starts to accumulate. Using the strong solution of ACV (1:1) toss down 3 cups of the mixture and run hot water over this from the kitchen tap. It helps to kill the odor as well as unclogging build up and disinfecting the drainage system.

Washing Machine

Cleaning the washing machine is easy if you just toss in a cupful of ACV (1:2) with the wash. It helps to clean up bits of calcification and disinfect all in one go.

Steam Iron

Cleaning your steam iron works on the same principle. Put a teaspoon of diluted (1:3) ACV in with the steam water and let it work away on the innards of the iron as you go through the pile of washing.

Appliances

Modern kitchens are often full of stainless steel appliances, and your bottle of strong ACV solution is great for bringing up a shine on stainless steel. It cuts through grease which may have splattered on the surfaces and prepares the metal for polishing up with a soft dry cloth afterwards.

Cutting Boards

Use your prepared spray bottle of 1:2 ACV for your cutting boards and don't forget to mark which board is for the onions!

Fridge/Freezer

The interior of your fridge or freezer will be disinfected and any fungal spores removed if you wipe it down regularly with your strong dilution of ACV.

Ice Trays

While you are busy in the fridge/freezer give those ice trays a wipe out after a soak in your sink full of diluted ACV (1:2)

Kettles etc.

Coffee makers and kettles can both benefit from a wipe-down to cleanse and a soak to de-scale in your 1:2 solution.

Bottles

Got bottles you want to keep, but their labels seem like they are stuck on with super glue. Try soaking in warm 1:2 ACV and leave overnight. It works out the stickiness.

Bathroom

Now moving to the bathroom as another room in the house that can do with some deep cleaning and freshening up. Remember that you can have your prepared bottles of strong ACV solution 1:1 or 1:2 concentrations depending if you have some industrial strength cleaning to do or if it is just the daily or weekly wipe down.

You can make them even more pleasant, as well as effective, by adding in drops of lovely essential oil to give the room a characteristic scent. Most manufacturers of cleaning products use lavender, lemon or pine scents, and we have come to associate them with 'clean' however you can just as easily use your own favorites. Try the crisp smell of bergamot, the floral delicacy of ylang-ylang or rose geranium or the round warmth of sandalwood. They are a bit different but can add subtly to the ambiance in your bathroom.

It's fun to experiment and see who in the family notices something different!

Makeup Brushes

Makeup brushes need a short weekly soak in your 1:2 solution of ACV to make them scrupulously clean for using on your face.   It is a wonderful non-toxic cleaner.

Toothbrush holder

While you do that, your Toothbrush holder can have a soak too.

Bathroom Ceramics

Your toilet, sink, and bath can all be wiped down with ACV solution to degrease and disinfect.

Shower Cubicle

However don't forget your showerhead, curtain and track will also really benefit from a good deep clean with 1:1 or 1:2 solution to get rid of mildew or fungal spores which may be lurking.

Dining Room

The dining room is often the place where we have candles. These look wonderful when they are lit but can disintegrate into runnels of wax which need to be removed by a solution of 1:2 ACV in the morning.

Lounge

Using your prepared bottle of 1:2 ACV spray your rugs to freshen them up and clean them. Let it dry then give the rugs a good shake and vacuum. That fusty smell should be gone then.

Wood Scratches

Wood scratches can be removed or at least improved by mixing ACV with olive oil. Half a cup of each and then applied with a soft cloth will bring up the wood beautifully. Great if the wood has drink rings, coffee stains, and sun faded bits on the surface.

Office

Electronics

Our daily lives are dominated by mobiles, cell phones, PC's, printers and other pieces of electronic equipment. These also need a wipe down with your 1:3 to keep them disinfected and mold free.

Ink

Ink stains soak away if you put a splash of ACV on them and let that soak in for 10 minutes. Then make a stiff paste with the ACV and cornstarch and rub into the stain. Dry the paste out and then wash off as normal.

Patio

Yeuk - Bird droppings all over the place again as our feathered friends come to roost or breed. Your 1:1 solution comes to the rescue, cleaning and disinfecting as you brush it over of the patio.

Garden Furniture

Garden furniture needs to have a good spring clean before it is ready for good company and the barbeque. Use your 1:2 ACV solution and wipe everything down. Gets rid of the dust and the germs, mildew, and fungus which may have accumulated over the winter.

In an ideal world you would have down this 'wipe down' in the Autumn as you put the furniture away for winter - but we aren't all quite as organised as that!

Garden

In the garden, a solution of ACV works as a weed killer, an insecticide, and a pesticide! Pretty useful, I think you'll agree!

Weed killer

As a weedkiller for species like dandelions try your industrial strength 1:1 ACV and apply it every day for a week or until you see the plant beginning to wilt. Don't water it accidentally. Just let the ACV soak down to the roots and begin to kill the plant.

Insect Trap

As an insect trap, it works wonderfully when you put some in a cup and let the aroma of the sweetish vinegar waft out to attract fruit flies and bugs galore. If you also mix the ACV with liquid dishwasher soap, the flies will die as they are attracted to the ACV but then damaged by the soap which interferes with their cell membranes. You can put this mixture in an old yogurt pot and punch a hole in the lid which they will find and crawl through.

Pesticide

Flowers and trees with pests can be sprayed with your 1:2 solution of ACV to discourage flying or fungal invasions.

Chapter 6 - Making your own ACV

Apple Cider Vinegar isn't particularly cheap to buy as it is usually sold from the local Natural Health food shop. Some supermarkets have it, but they tend to sell it in a pasteurized form which means there is no 'mother' in it. In the States 1 quart ACV = $5+ but the good news is that you can easily make 4 times that (1 gallon) at home for even less!

To do this let's go back to basics and remember the history of our amazing ACV. It started as just apple juice, crushed for the folks during the harvest as they gathered in the apples. It made a wonderfully sweet, refreshing drink. Then, when there was some juice left people found that it began to ferment if it was left to gather up the tiny micro-organisms of yeasts and spores in the air. Left to itself it began to form into alcohol and the first ciders were made. The taste depended on the amount of fermentation allowed and the taste of the original apples in it. From then - if there was any cider left! - people went on to discover that if it was left alone even longer, the microscopic yeasts began to absorb and feed off the sugars and alcohol and turn them into vinegar.

So to begin your brewing of your very own ACV start with:

Getting together a wide-mouthed gallon jar. Preferably get a glass or ceramic one as the final vinegar would interact with plastic.

Get a piece of cheesecloth large enough to cover the mouth of the jar. An old clean tea towel would be great.

A long spoon for stirring.

A sharp knife for chopping the apples.

Colander to strain the liquid - or a larger piece of cheesecloth.

5 large apples - try to get a variety of apples at your local organic greengrocer. You ideally want 3 sweet tasting apples, 2 sharp or 1 sharp and one bitter.

1 cup local honey

Filtered water

Chop up the apples into small pieces, keep the peel on.

Half fill a 1-gallon jar with the apples.

Put the honey into the 1-gallon jar and cover with water until the water is just 2" from the rim of the jar. (Reminder: Apples to about half way up the jar and water to 2 inches below top).

Cover with cheesecloth and leave on kitchen surface for 1 week and give the mixture a stir a couple of times/day.

After the week is up strain the mixture and from the smell, you will find that you now have a flat cider!

Cover again with cheesecloth, put the jar in a dark place and leave it alone for 3 or 4 weeks. You will notice the 'Mother' floating around like strands of a jellyfish when you open it up. This is a great sign as you know that the alcohol has been converted to vinegar.

You have now got apple cider vinegar. Yay! Enjoy.

Goodbye and Good Natural Health

We hope you have enjoyed this book on Apple Cider Vinegar and that you will start using it as part of your cleaning arsenal, or health boosting remedies and beauty routines.

Natural health is a way of life and a wonderful way to keep you and your family as healthy as possible. Everyone will be able to fight off viruses when the winter comes, stave off allergic responses as spring pollens float into the air and know how to take care of themselves if they have stings and bites from our winged 'friends' in Summer.

We have a series of ebooks on various Natural Health Remedies and how to enhance your life through Mindful practices. Our wish for you is to live happily and healthily in the present moment and to enjoy every moment of your life. You are always welcome to get in touch with us, and we look forward to helping you.

www.YourWellnessBooks.com

Until next time

Be Beautiful, Be Healthy, Be Happy…

I hope you will enjoy your holistic health and beauty journey!

I hope to "see" you in my next book.

Love,

Cassia Albinson

In the meantime, check out more of our books below:

www.YourWellnessBooks.com

www.ingramcontent.com/pod-product-compliance
Lightning Source LLC
Chambersburg PA
CBHW041218030426
42336CB00023B/3380